The Library of Sexual Health™

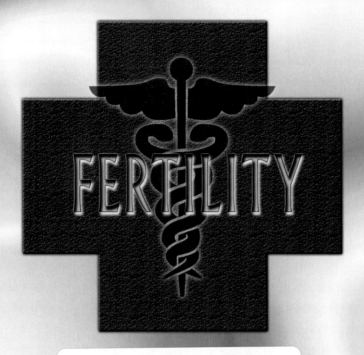

FERTILITY

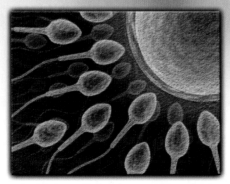

MICHAEL R. WILSON

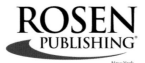

ROSEN
PUBLISHING®

New York

Published in 2009 by The Rosen Publishing Group, Inc.
29 East 21st Street, New York, NY 10010

Library of Congress Cataloging-in-Publication Data

Wilson, Michael R., 1967–
Fertility / Michael R. Wilson.—1st ed.
     p. cm.—(the library of sexual health)
Includes bibliographical references and index.
ISBN-13: 978-1-4358-5063-7 (lib. bdg.)
1. Human reproductive technology. 2. Fertility, Human. 3. Infertility.
I. Title.
RG133.5.W545 2009
618.1'78—dc22

                                                      2008017895

Manufactured in Malaysia

CONTENTS

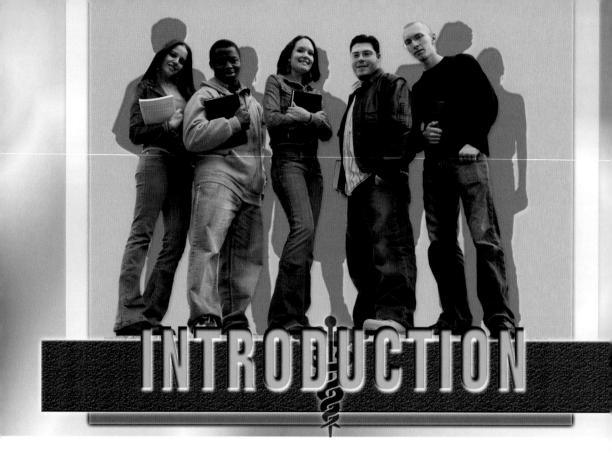

INTRODUCTION

With nearly seven billion people on the planet, and hundreds of thousands more being born every day, it may sound strange to single out one birth as particularly important. But when Louise Joy Brown was delivered in Oldham, England, on July 25, 1978, everything changed. Brown was the world's very first baby to be conceived using in vitro fertilization.

In vitro fertilization, or IVF, is a laboratory technique that involves surgically removing a woman's eggs from her ovaries and combining them with a man's sperm. Once the eggs are fertilized, they are transferred into the woman's uterus. They can also be transferred to a woman other than the one who donated the eggs.

Why would anyone go to such great lengths just to have kids? The answer has to do with fertility, or the ability to conceive and carry a pregnancy to birth. Most people take fertility for granted. When they decide to have children, they just go ahead and do it. It may take a month or two to become pregnant, but it's usually not a big deal.

Sometimes, however, fertility is not so straightforward. Many people are infertile—for one reason or another, they can't have children naturally. In the case of Louise Joy Brown, her mother had a physical problem with her fallopian tubes, the narrow passageways between the ovaries and the uterus. A blockage in her tubes prevented her eggs from becoming fertilized.

Brown's parents decided to try what was then a cutting-edge technique to achieve artificial fertilization. They are believed to be the first people in the world to succeed in having a child this way.

Fertility is an important aspect of who we are in so many ways—physically, socially, and psychologically. For this reason, infertility can be extremely difficult. Even though it's not life threatening by itself, infertility can become a serious condition requiring medical attention.

Good sexual health is key to fertility and infertility, as the human reproductive tract must be healthy for conception to occur. Overall health, too, is important to fertility. The human body is incredibly complicated, and a single problem in one part of the body can have negative effects throughout the body.

This book is about fertility and infertility. It starts off by providing an overview of normal human fertility and reproduction. Then, it discusses the possible problems that can lead to infertility. Later chapters go through some of the more common treatments for infertility and ways that individuals and couples cope with being infertile. There is also discussion of certain things that you can do to maintain good reproductive health and, hopefully, reduce your risk of becoming infertile.

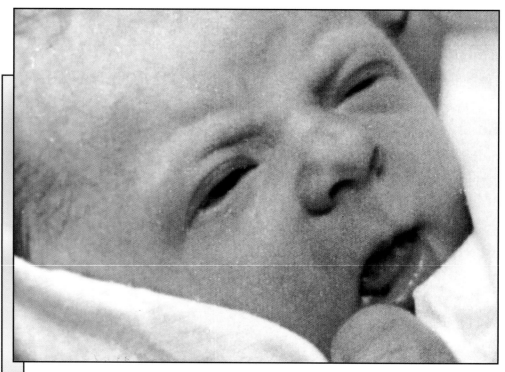

The world's first "test tube baby" was Louise Joy Brown *(above)*. In 1978, she was delivered by Caesarian section at Oldham General Hospital in Lancashire, England.

Use this book any way you like—as a source of information for a school report, for example, or even for ideas that you can use in your own life. If you know someone who is infertile and is having trouble coping, then maybe this book will help you come up with a few ways that you can help.

When you're through reading, take a few minutes to look at the additional resources listed at the end of this book. You'll find other books, useful Web sites, helpful organizations, and additional references. Taken together, they should supply all the information you will need to become fully educated about fertility, infertility, and sexual health.

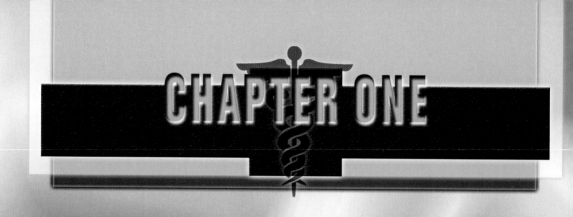

CHAPTER ONE

The Biology of Fertility

I n order to understand infertility, you should first have a good idea of what it means to be fertile. You should also know about the biological and physical processes that have to take place in order for fertilization to occur. So, buckle your seatbelt. It's time for a talk about sex, eggs, sperm, and babies.

LET'S TALK ABOUT SEX

It's simple, really. For fertilization to occur, you need sperm from a man and an egg from a woman. The sperm and egg can be introduced to each other naturally (through sexual intercourse) or artificially (through assistive reproductive technology). Either way, without sperm and an egg, there is no baby. This section of the book on normal fertility will discuss fertilization the way it occurs naturally.

A man and a woman have sexual intercourse. At some point during sex, the man ejaculates and millions of sperm enter the woman's vagina. (The typical healthy man produces more than four hundred million sperm in his testes every day.) Most of these sperm die soon after ejaculation. Others spill out of the vagina, while some are weak or unhealthy and don't go anywhere.

Strong sperm, meanwhile, start swimming. Carried in semen, they climb up through the vaginal canal, through the cervix, and into the uterus. A couple hundred or more make it all the way to the fallopian tubes, which connect the woman's uterus to her ovaries. But hold on. We've got the sperm, even if it's just a few hundred, hanging out in the fallopian tube. What's happening on the woman's side of things?

A woman's menstrual cycle (period) is controlled by hormones that occur naturally in her body. These hormones lead to the production of eggs in her ovaries. (*Ova* is Latin for "eggs.") Women normally have two walnut-sized ovaries. The eggs grow in tiny sacs called follicles.

Sometime around the middle of that cycle (day fourteen), ovulation occurs. A follicle breaks open and an egg is released. If more than one egg is released, as sometimes happens, then there is potential for a multiple pregnancy—twins, triplets, etc. Once an egg is released from an ovary, it begins to travel down the fallopian tube toward the uterus, an organ also known as the womb. For the next twenty-four hours or so, the egg is available for fertilization.

If the egg does not get fertilized, then the woman will menstruate. The egg travels to the uterus and is shed from the body during the bleeding that signals the beginning of a woman's period.

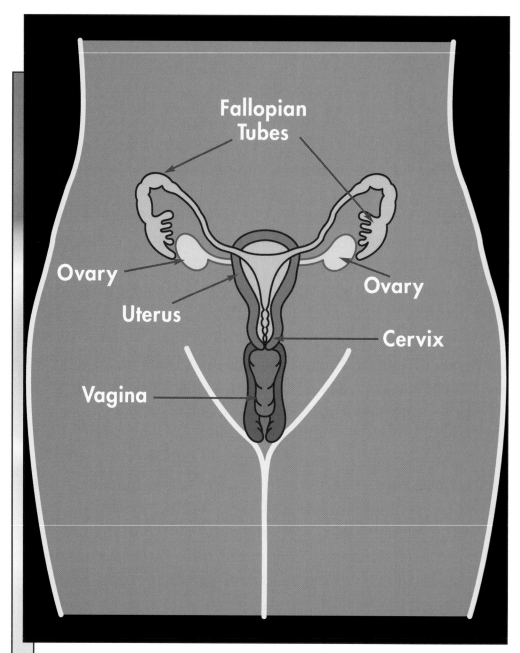

A woman's reproductive organs are located in her lower abdomen, or pelvis. All the organs shown here play important roles in fertility.

But we're talking about fertilization, so let's go back to that "available" egg. As mentioned earlier, of the millions of sperm in a man's ejaculate, relatively few make it as far as the fallopian tubes. If the timing is just right, then those that do make it will find the egg in waiting. More often, however, because ovulation occurs just once a month, there is no egg in the fallopian tubes. Sperm can survive in the female reproductive tract for up to seventy-two hours. If they do not come across an egg during that time, then fertilization can't take place.

FERTILIZATION AND GROWTH

Let's assume there is an egg available for fertilization. Only one sperm can fertilize it. The others are out of luck. Fertilization takes place when that one sperm meets and then binds with the egg. This combination of a man's sperm with a woman's egg creates a one-celled zygote. The moment of fertilization is also known as conception. Pregnancy is defined as the time of conception until birth.

The one-celled zygote now moves in the direction of the uterus. From here, to greatly simplify, a series of cellular processes will combine the chromosomes from the sperm and egg. This ensures that the future offspring has genetic material from both parents. Cell division begins, and before long, the original one-celled zygote grows into the millions and then billions of cells that form a human being.

The dividing zygote travels down the fallopian tube to the uterus, a distance of about two to four inches. There,

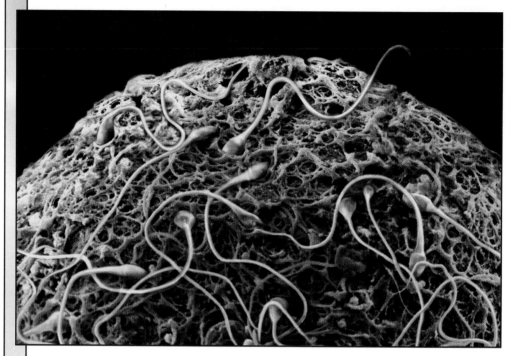

This scanning electron micrograph shows several sperm swarming over an egg. Ultimately, only one sperm will penetrate the egg to fertilize it.

the zygote nestles into the inner lining of the uterus, called the endometrium. Over time, the endometrium grows thicker, providing a protective, nutrient-rich place for the embryo to grow.

The developing human is called an embryo from the third week to the eighth week of pregnancy. It's called a fetus from the ninth week until birth, and it's called an infant after delivery. Delivery takes place when the baby is pushed from its place in the uterus through the cervix and out the vagina.

Ten Facts About Fertility

1. Number of women in the United States between the ages of fifteen and forty-four with impaired ability to have children: 6.1 million.

2. Number of women in the United States who have ever used infertility services: 9.2 million.

3. Number of married couples in the United States that are infertile: 2.1 million.

4. About one-third of infertile women are between the ages of thirty-five and forty-four.

5. Infertility affects all races and socioeconomic groups equally.

6. Those in higher socioeconomic groups (wealthier people) use infertility services much more often than poorer people.

7. In vitro fertilization is partially responsible for the recent 70 percent increase in multiple pregnancies (twins, triplets, etc.) in the United States.

8. Of the millions of sperm released at ejaculation, only one can fertilize any single egg.

9. At least three million American youth contract an STD each year.

10. An estimated thirty million American men have erectile dysfunction, a common cause of infertility.

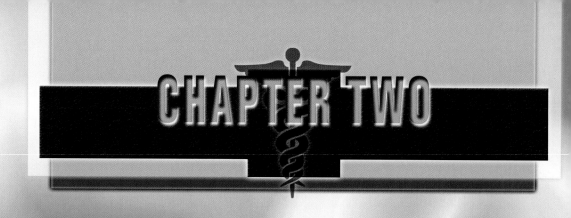

Infertility and Its Causes

N ow that you have a decent idea as to how conception works, let's consider the many things that can go wrong, leading to infertility. A woman who is infertile is either unable to get pregnant or, once pregnant, unable to carry that pregnancy to term. A man who is infertile is unable to impregnate a fertile woman after at least a year of trying. A couple typically isn't diagnosed with a fertility problem until they've tried to conceive for at least six months.

Some women can't get pregnant because they have reached menopause. In other words, because of the natural aging process, they no longer produce eggs for fertilization. Technically, these women are not considered infertile; they are simply no longer of normal childbearing age. Menopause usually takes place around the age of fifty, at the end of a natural decline in hormone production that begins in the mid-thirties.

Infertility can occur because of a reproductive problem with the man, the woman, or both. Sometimes, it's due to

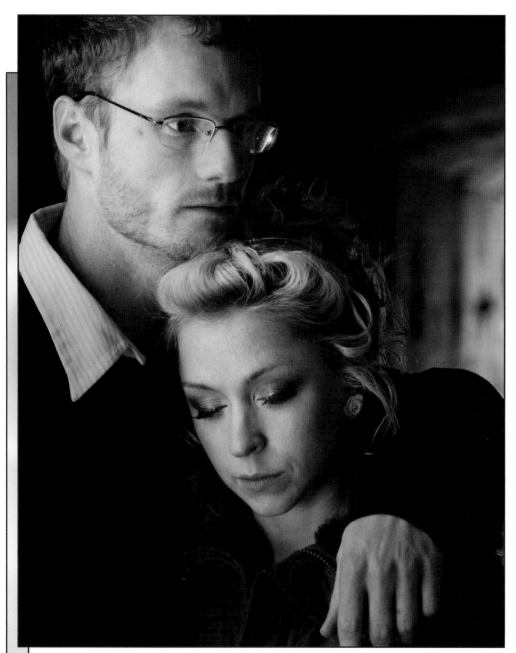

Infertility is a real emotional burden on people who want to have children.
Fortunately, most couples find a way to conceive and have children in the end.

a hormone problem. For example, if a man is not getting adequate testosterone production from his testes, then he may have a low sperm count. An infertile woman may have low levels of the hormones LH (luteinizing hormone) and FSH (follicle stimulating hormone). Those two hormones are required for normal egg production and ovulation.

Infertility may also be the result of a wide range of medical or physical conditions that harm the reproductive system. For instance, some women develop knotty, fibrous growths in their fallopian tubes that block passage of a fertilized egg. Others may experience such intense pain during intercourse that they are unable to get impregnated. Some men can't hold an erection long enough to have sexual intercourse, or they ejaculate before intercourse can occur. Others fail to produce enough semen in their ejaculate. If a man has testicular cancer, then he may need surgery to remove the diseased testes. (Men may still be fertile if only one testis is removed, however.) Ovarian cancer might make it necessary to remove a woman's ovaries, making ovulation impossible.

LOOKING AT RISKS

Often, infertility is just a game of chance. Sometimes, people lack the genes required for adequate levels of sperm production or for any kind of egg production. A genetic condition known as congenital absence of the vas deferens, for instance, allows a man to produce sperm but not to transfer that sperm from his testes to his ejaculate. Without sperm in the ejaculate, there is no natural way to send it to an egg for fertilization. Another condition called Klinefelter's syndrome results in the man having an extra X chromosome. This leads to poor testicular development and low or no sperm production.

Another contributor to infertility is age. As people get older, their bodies wear down. Along with the visible wear and tear (wrinkling, graying hair, etc.), there are also substantial changes taking place internally. Sperm quality decreases in men beginning in their twenties. As mentioned above, women's egg production stops with menopause, around age fifty.

Poor diet, alcohol and drug abuse, smoking, and taking certain medications can all contribute to the decline of reproductive health and eventual infertility. Environmental toxins in the air, water, and soil are also believed to play a role. And then, of course, there are sexually transmitted diseases (STDs).

CAUSES OF INFERTILITY

Here's a quick rundown on some of the more common causes of infertility, beginning with STDs.

STDs 101

Among the biggest threats to fertility are sexually transmitted diseases. You've probably heard about STDs before, most likely in sex ed. Sexually transmitted diseases are spread through sexual contact, including vaginal sex, anal sex, oral sex, and even kissing. Sometimes, genital contact is all that is necessary for an STD to spread from one person to another. Millions of people contract STDs every year. According to the U.S. Centers for Disease Control and Prevention (CDC), three million American youths ages ten to nineteen are among them.

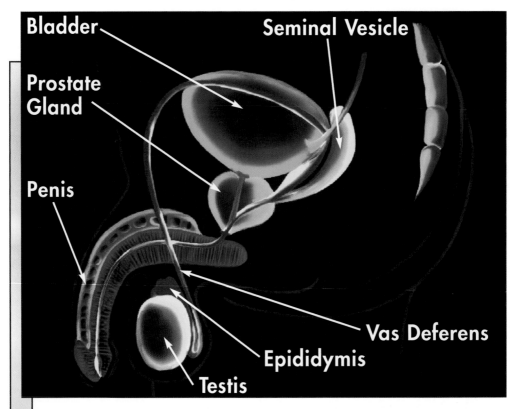

Bladder

Seminal Vesicle

Prostate Gland

Penis

Vas Deferens

Epididymis

Testis

This computer illustration shows the male reproductive organs. Various sexually transmitted diseases can damage one or more of these organs, leading to infertility.

There are many different kinds of STDs. HIV/AIDS is the best known and the deadliest. Others include chlamydia, syphilis, genital warts and genital herpes, gonorrhea, trichomoniasis, and hepatitis B. Teens have particularly high rates of chlamydia and gonorrhea, both of which can cause health complications that compromise fertility. Among women, a primary STD-related cause of infertility is PID, or pelvic inflammatory disease (see below). Among men, repeated STD infection may lead to a condition called epididymitis, which is inflammation of the epididymis, the tube that carries semen from the testicles. Because these conditions typically develop over many years of STD exposure, people who are infected with STDs in their teenage years are at particular risk.

Pelvic Inflammatory Disease and Fallopian Tube Damage

Pelvic inflammatory disease, or PID, is a disease of the female reproductive tract. It is caused by pathogenic (harmful) bacteria. The bacteria enter the reproductive tract through the vagina, most commonly during sexual intercourse. Most women who get PID get it when they contract a bacterial STD such as gonorrhea or chlamydia. In some cases, the bacteria may be introduced during surgical procedures or other activities that expose the vagina to contamination.

PID can create all kinds of problems for a woman. One of the biggest problems is chronic pain, usually caused by the buildup of scar tissue in the fallopian tubes. The scar tissue develops because of the bacterial infestation. It is the body's natural response to an unwanted intruder. Scar tissue is very stiff and bumpy. If it builds up too much, then it can block the fallopian tubes entirely. If this happens, then eggs may not be able to travel from the ovaries, where they're produced, to the uterus. Fertilization becomes impossible, and infertility results.

Most women with PID can be cured of the disease if it's detected early and treated right away. Treatment includes taking antibiotics, which are special drugs designed to fight bacteria.

Even though PID is treatable, 20 percent of women who get PID do eventually become infertile. Infertility is most prevalent among those who get PID more than once. This is an all-too-common occurrence, especially in women with multiple sex partners who have unprotected sex.

Polycystic Ovary Syndrome

Polycystic ovary syndrome, or PCOS, occurs when a woman's ovaries develop hard, lumpy cysts. By themselves, the cysts do not cause infertility. However, the cysts, along with other PCOS symptoms, result in poor ovulation.

Under normal circumstances, eggs develop in follicles within the ovaries until they are ready for release. In women with PCOS, the eggs sometimes remain stuck within the follicles. Or, if the eggs are released, they often

Teens, Sex, Pregnancy, and STDs

Any discussion about fertility must at least make mention of teens and pregnancy. There is some good news in this regard. According to the Federal Interagency Forum on Child and Family Statistics, the teen birth rate in 2005 hit an all-time low. Fewer teens are having sex, and those who do have sex are using barrier forms of birth control such as condoms. Use of a condom not only helps to prevent unwanted pregnancies, but it also protects against sexually transmitted diseases (STDs) that can lead to serious health problems.

Still, hundreds of thousands of teenage girls continue to get pregnant every year, while millions contract STDs. The consequences of an unintended pregnancy are obvious. When an individual gets an STD, on the other hand, a number of things can happen—anything from a relatively harmless skin rash to infertility, AIDS, and death. Studies have shown that nearly 50 percent of new STD cases every year occur among those who are between the ages of fifteen and twenty-four.

Even though they are dropping, the rates of unplanned pregnancies and STDs in the United States are still too high. Some experts think the high rates have a lot to do with American society and culture. After all, sex appears to be everywhere—in the movies, on television, in magazine advertisements, and online. When it looks like everyone around you is having sex, it's easy to think that you should be having sex, too.

Meanwhile, sex education in the United States is seriously lagging when compared to that in other developed countries. "Abstinence-only" education, for example, does not include talk about condoms and how they can be an effective means of STD prevention. Many experts believe that sex education must include an open discussion about all things sex-related in order to better reflect the reality of our times.

Will all this change in the future? Probably. It takes time, however, and until then, the key thing for any teenager to think about is this: the decision to begin having sex is an intensely personal one. The potential consequences of a mistake are too high for it to be otherwise.

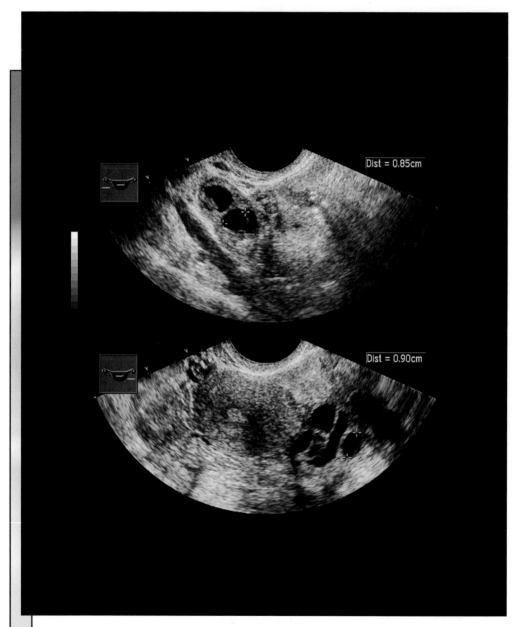

Ultrasound scans show the presence of multiple cysts (black, round shapes) in a woman's ovary. Most ovarian cysts are harmless and disappear over time.

are not healthy enough to be fertilized. In some cases, fertilization may take place, but then the fertilized egg doesn't successfully make the journey from the fallopian tube to the uterus. Without implantation in the uterus, the fertilized egg will not receive the nutrients that it needs to grow and develop into an embryo, and the pregnancy will end. An estimated 10 percent of women who are of child-bearing age have PCOS. However, many of these women have no idea that they have the condition because its symptoms can be difficult to recognize.

PCOS is believed to be hereditary and is caused by hormone imbalances in the body. Many women with PCOS have high levels of the hormone insulin, which in turn can lead to increased testosterone production. Testosterone is a male hormone, but healthy women also produce it in small quantities. Ovarian cysts may result when the woman's body produces too much testosterone and too little of the female hormones estrogen and progesterone. There is no cure for PCOS, but symptoms may be treated with medication, and women with PCOS can lead otherwise healthy lives.

Endometriosis

If a woman's uterine lining—her endometrium—grows outside of her uterus, then she is said to have endometriosis. Endometriosis leads to scar tissue development, which in turn can prevent the ovaries, uterus, and fallopian tubes from functioning as they should. Some studies show that as many as 30 percent of women going for infertility treatment show signs of endometriosis.

Premature Ovarian Failure

Premature ovarian failure is also known as early menopause. A woman with this condition stops producing eggs many years before she normally would (around age fifty). Early menopause can be caused by smoking, harsh cancer treatments such as radiation therapy, and certain diseases.

ERECTILE DYSFUNCTION

If a man consistently cannot get or maintain an erection long enough to have sexual intercourse, then he has erectile dysfunction. Also known as impotence, it occurs when not enough blood flows into the penis to make it hard. Without an erection, it is difficult or impossible to have sex.

It is estimated that thirty million American men have erectile dysfunction. The condition has several different causes, including everything from stress and depression to drug and alcohol abuse or the side effects of prescription medication. Erectile dysfunction may also be caused by physical problems or trauma.

Low testosterone levels are often a factor in erectile dysfunction. Testosterone is the hormone responsible for sperm production, but it also plays a major role in a man's ability to become sexually aroused. With very low testosterone, getting an erection may be extremely difficult or even impossible. Because testosterone levels drop off naturally with age, elderly men often develop erectile dysfunction. Low testosterone can also result from an injury to the testes, from treatment for testicular cancer, or from genetic problems.

SPERM PROBLEMS

Low or poor-quality sperm production is another common cause of infertility. Low sperm production can result from inadequate testosterone. Poor-quality sperm, or sperm that are unable to fertilize an egg, may be attributed to various causes, including drug and alcohol abuse, poor nutrition, or general poor health.

When it comes to fertility, it's important for a man to have adequate sperm production. Only a very small percentage of the millions of sperm sent into the vagina at ejaculation even make it to the egg. If a man's sperm count is limited, then the chances that his sperm will successfully fertilize an egg decrease dramatically.

It's also important that sperm be strong and healthy. They must be fully developed, with tails that can propel them deep into the female reproductive tract. Sperm that are not healthy stand little chance of completing the long journey to a waiting egg. Even if they do make it, they may struggle to penetrate the egg to achieve fertilization.

UNDESCENDED TESTICLE

Undescended testicle is a problem that occurs during fetal development when one or both of the testes fail to drop from the abdomen into the scrotum. Usually, this condition is repaired before one year of age. If it's not fixed, then the higher body temperature within the abdomen can

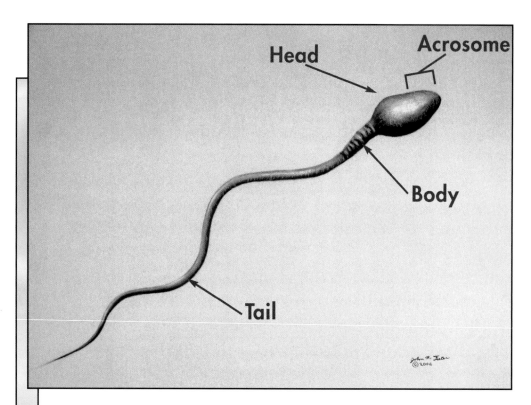

This illustration of a sperm cell clearly shows its large head, which carries the father's genetic material. The acrosome, at the tip of the head, is designed to penetrate the outer layers of an egg. The sperm's long tail is also called a flagellum.

prevent the testis (or testes) from producing adequate sperm. Fortunately, fertility should not be affected if there is a normal-functioning testis. Also, there is some evidence that fertility is not adversely affected if the testis is "brought down" before age eleven.

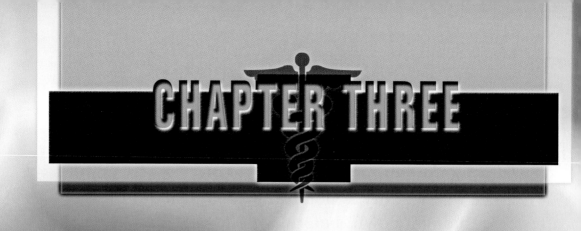

CHAPTER THREE

Staying Fertile

V ery often, there is nothing one can do to prevent infertility. You're born with the genes you have, after all, and sometimes the luck of the draw just isn't that lucky. Still, beyond the genetic lottery and the natural decline in fertility that comes with age, individuals can take certain steps to stay fertile. Regular medical check-ups, for instance, are a great way to monitor overall health, detect problems early, and avoid conditions that might compromise fertility. Making good choices when it comes to relationships and sex is also important. Finally, maintaining a healthy lifestyle is critical to overall good health.

STD PREVENTION

Sexually transmitted diseases such as chlamydia and gonorrhea are common causes of infertility. So, prevention of these diseases is critical. The key to STD prevention is education. If you know how to protect yourself, then you drastically reduce your chances of contracting an STD. What do you need to know?

First of all, you can get an STD the very first time you have sex. It doesn't matter who your partner is, since it's impossible to know for sure that a partner is STD-free. It's important to ask any sexual partner whether he or she has been tested for STDs and what the results were. If you've had sexual relations in the past, then it's also important to be tested yourself. After that, the key to prevention is either practicing abstinence or using protection. It's also important to maintain a mutually monogamous (one partner only) relationship. Having sex with more than one person greatly increases your chances of getting an STD.

Abstinence means not having sex at all. For some people, this is easy. They don't want to have sex and they're not ready for sex, so they don't have it. For others, peer pressure makes things more difficult. It can help to have close friends who feel the same way that you do about sex.

Protection, when it comes to STD prevention, usually involves condoms. The latex condom is a barrier form of birth control. Unlike oral forms of birth control such as the Pill, a condom physically blocks sperm from entering the vagina. It's also effective at limiting the spread of STDs. Still, no form of protection works all of the time.

If you ever find yourself short on STD information, then ask your doctor or a school nurse for help. Either one will be happy to answer any questions you may have.

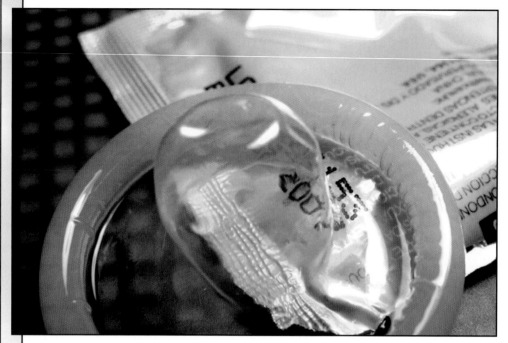

Condoms are a type of barrier protection. They help prevent pregnancy, and they also block the spread of most STDs during sexual contact.

LIFESTYLE CHANGES

Sometimes, infertility is related to poor overall health, which in turn can be improved by making simple changes to one's lifestyle. Taking steps to reduce stress, for example, can significantly reduce blood pressure, improve sleep, and help improve one's sense of well-being. Stress reduction often involves a reassessment of priorities—putting more emphasis on exercise and personal time and less on money problems, job requirements, and things that are out of one's control.

Diet is another important component of good overall health. A diet full of whole foods, fruits, and vegetables and without too much added sugar, salt, or artificial ingredients is a sure way to keep weight down, muscle mass up, and all body systems operating at full speed.

Needless to say, exercise is also important. Most experts recommend exercising at least three times a week for half an hour a day. More exercise is better, especially the activities that boost your heart rate for extended periods. Get your pulse up, and you're bound to see improvements in overall health.

Finally, it goes without saying that use of illegal drugs and alcohol can damage your overall health in general and your reproductive health specifically. Pregnant women in particular should never smoke or drink, as doing so can harm the developing fetus.

Some men with low sperm counts or poor-quality sperm have seen improvements by making simple changes to the clothes they wear. Clothes that are too tight around the crotch can increase the testicular temperature and kill sperm. Especially among those who are actively trying to conceive, it's a good idea to wear loose-fitting clothing.

Some studies have also shown that the very hot temperatures common in hot tubs and saunas can be detrimental to sperm health. There is even speculation that the heat generated in the crotch area during long-distance bicycle rides can hurt sperm quality. This link is unproven, however, and most health experts agree the

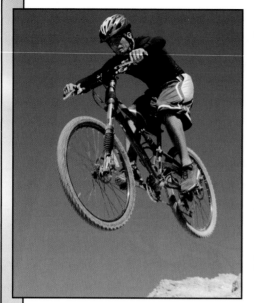

This guy obviously has skills, but how will he land? When riding a bike, be careful to avoid serious trauma to the testicles that can cause infertility.

cardiovascular and muscular benefits of bicycle riding far outweigh any risk to reproductive health.

ENVIRONMENTAL CONCERNS

Toxic chemicals in the environment can cause infertility, so it only makes sense to do everything that you can to avoid them. One way to keep chemical exposure to a minimum is by eating food that has been produced without the use of pesticides or herbicides. Look for organic food labels on store shelves and at local markets.

Other simple ways to keep chemical exposure down include installing a filter on your water tap, avoiding painting in unventilated rooms, not smoking or going near people who smoke, staying away from polluting cars and buses, never burning plastic, and avoiding the use of chemical-based household cleaners. There are countless other sources of chemical exposure that you should avoid. Just keep your eyes open and think. If it looks, smells, or tastes toxic, then it probably is.

Myths and Facts

MYTH: Infertile people must have done something wrong—like taken illegal drugs, drunk too much, or eaten something that was bad for them—that caused their infertility.
FACT: Unhealthy lifestyles can lead to infertility, but infertility is usually due to some other factor. Some people are born infertile. Others have physical problems, diseases, or conditions that prevent fertilization from occurring.

MYTH: Infertility is a woman's problem.
FACT: More than half the time, it's either the man's problem or a combination of problems with the man and the woman. And other times, it's impossible to tell where the problem lies. The woman may be the one who ultimately gives birth, but that doesn't mean infertility is a problem all her own. Remember, it takes two to tango.

MYTH: If you're having trouble getting pregnant, then there's a good chance you're infertile.
FACT: Not quite. Many couples have trouble achieving pregnancy because of timing issues. They may not be having sex during the right time in the woman's cycle. For fertilization to occur, there must be sperm in the woman's body around the time she ovulates. Many couples find that achieving pregnancy takes a long time. The commonly accepted definition of infertility, after all, is the inability to conceive after a full year of trying.

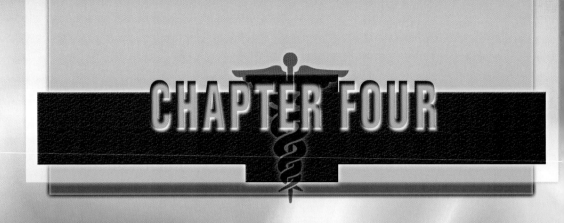

CHAPTER FOUR

Diagnosis and Treatment

Most people have no idea that they have fertility issues until they try to have children. If conception doesn't occur right away, then it's usually no cause for concern. After all, many couples go through months of trying before they succeed. However, there may be a problem if they still can't get pregnant after trying for a year. At this point, most doctors would suggest coming in for examination.

INFERTILITY DIAGNOSIS

Technically, a couple that fails to conceive after one year is medically infertile. In practice, however, it's more complicated than that. While they may be "infertile," fertility may be well within their reach, even without using artificial methods in order to achieve it.

Any individuals or couple seeking medical help for infertility will first be asked about their general health. The doctor will take a medical history and ask questions about everything from past health conditions and surgeries to sexual history and practices. Following that, the doctor will conduct a physical exam, including an exam of the pelvic area to look for any obvious signs of a problem. Blood work may be asked for, in which case blood will be drawn and sent to a lab for analysis. One thing a doctor might look for in the blood test is a hormone imbalance. He or she might also want to analyze blood sugar levels, cholesterol, and other indicators of overall health.

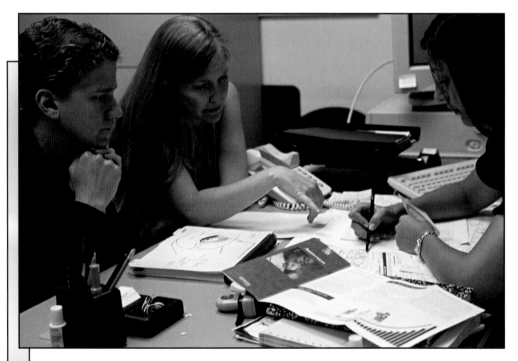

Many couples seek outside help for their infertility. Trained professionals offer everything from genetic counseling to options for medical treatment.

The doctor may decide to use imaging technology to take a look inside the body. Common imaging techniques include ultrasound, CT scan, and MRI. Each of these noninvasive and completely painless procedures produces detailed images of reproductive organs or other parts of the body that may be responsible for the fertility problem. Testing may be conducted on the man, the woman, or both, depending on the situation.

There may also be questions about the couple's attempts at pregnancy. Many individuals, for example, have no idea that timing plays a crucial role in achieving pregnancy. If sexual intercourse does not take place within a specific window of time during the woman's monthly cycle, then the odds of getting pregnant drop dramatically.

FERTILITY TREATMENT

Infertility, while challenging for many people, is not life threatening. Once an individual or couple is diagnosed as infertile, they have several choices to consider. How they decide to proceed may depend on anything from health insurance and financial resources to their religious practices and convictions. Ultimately, two-thirds of couples treated for infertility go on to become fertile and have children.

Fertility treatment can be very complicated and emotionally uprooting. One approach to infertility is medical treatment. Some people undergo surgery to correct problems with their reproductive system. Others need to take synthetic (human-produced) hormones or special medications. Hormone therapy may include injections of testosterone, LH, or FSH until sperm production or ovulation is adequate.

Sometimes, surgery may be required to remove a hormone-disrupting tumor from the body. If surgery is successful, then there is a good chance that fertility will be restored as an individual's hormone levels come back into balance.

For some infertile couples, the best option is to use assistive reproductive technology. The various techniques involve artificial or partially artificial procedures to fertilize an egg and implant it in the uterus. Below are a few of the more commonly used assistive reproductive techniques.

Artificial Insemination

With artificial insemination (AI), sperm is taken from a man and injected with a syringe into a woman's vagina. If a couple is trying to get pregnant and the man is known to have viable (healthy) sperm, then artificial insemination with his sperm may improve their chances of success. Sperm may also be taken from a sperm bank. Sperm banks are businesses that collect sperm from donors, freeze it, and then store it for future use. Couples or individuals can then purchase the sperm for use in artificial insemination.

In Vitro Fertilization (IVF)

As mentioned in the introduction to this book, in vitro fertilization involves the surgical transfer of fertilized eggs into a woman's uterus. The procedure involves removing eggs from a woman's ovaries and then fertilizing them in a laboratory with a man's sperm. (*In vitro* is Latin for "within the glass"; the fertilization actually takes place in a laboratory petri dish.) The sperm can come from the same man who intends to serve as the father of the child, or it may come from an outside donor. Likewise, the eggs may come from the woman hoping to conceive or from an egg donor.

Egg Donors

Women who give the eggs produced in their ovaries to other women who need them are called egg donors. Egg donation allows women who can't produce eggs, or who don't produce healthy eggs, the opportunity to have children. The egg removal is fairly simple. Fertility drugs (synthetic hormones) are given to the donor to induce superovulation, or ovulation of multiple eggs. Once ovulation occurs, minor surgery is performed to remove the eggs from the ovaries. The eggs are then taken to the lab and mixed with sperm. If fertilization

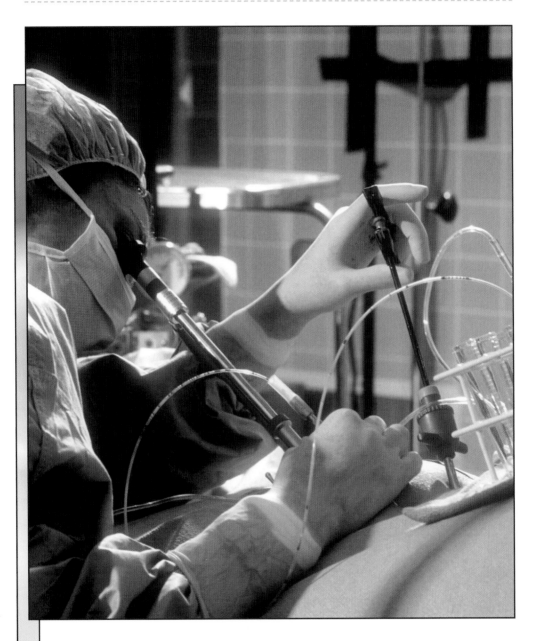

In vitro fertilization requires minor surgery to transfer the fertilized egg to the woman's uterus. This doctor is performing such a procedure, called a laparoscopy.

The Challenge of Multiple Births

One problem, so to speak, of in vitro fertilization is how often the procedure results in the birth of not just one healthy baby but in twins, triplets, quadruplets, and even quintuplets. The process typically involves transferring more than one embryo from the lab to the uterus in order to increase the chances of success. Usually only one embryo, if any, survives. But there's a far greater chance of a multiple pregnancy following in vitro fertilization than there is through normal fertilization following sexual intercourse. In fact, the birth rate of twins in the United States has increased by 70 percent since in vitro fertilization was first introduced, while other multiple births have increased drastically as well.

So, what's the problem? After all, anyone who tries in vitro fertilization must want to get pregnant. The more babies, the better, right? Well, maybe. As with most things in life, it's not as clear-cut as that. In fact, multiple pregnancies are more dangerous than normal pregnancies. Carrying multiple babies at once can be a physical strain on the mother. It can also lead to low-weight and high-risk births.

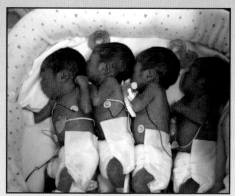

Since the first in vitro birth in 1978, infertility treatments have made multiple births much more common.

Fertility clinics worldwide are now trying to reduce their rates of multiple pregnancies. They are using new technologies that allow them to transfer fewer embryos (or even one embryo) at once while maintaining a high fertility success rate. The technique, called single embryo transfer, involves close laboratory analysis of developing embryos to determine which ones stand the greatest chance of survival.

Some people want twins from in vitro fertilization. The procedure costs many thousands of dollars, so some think it makes sense to get all of the childbearing done at once. Nevertheless, single embryo transfer is increasingly popular, and the multiple-pregnancy rate should therefore decrease over time.

occurs, then the fertilized eggs are implanted in the mother-to-be.

There are many requirements that prospective egg donors must meet before they can undergo the egg removal procedure. Typically, donors must be at least twenty-one years old and no older than thirty-five. (Studies indicate that after age thirty-five, there is an increased risk that donated eggs will have chromosomal or other defects.) Prospective donors must also take various tests designed to make sure that they are both physically and psychologically ready for the process. A gynecological exam, medical history, blood tests, ultrasound, STD testing, and even genetic testing are all standard. Psychological screening is typically conducted to weed out donors who may be donating out of a desperate need for money or who may end up feeling excessively attached to any future children they bear.

Matching up donors with women who need eggs is another component of many egg donor programs. The matching process raises certain ethical issues, or questions about what is right or wrong. Some companies maintain catalog-type guides to the donors that they have available. Egg buyers can browse these guides as they search for just the right match. For instance, they might look closely at donor heritage, intelligence, education, physical abilities, and other outward signs of talent that might indicate their ability to produce a particularly "qualified" egg.

OTHER SOLUTIONS

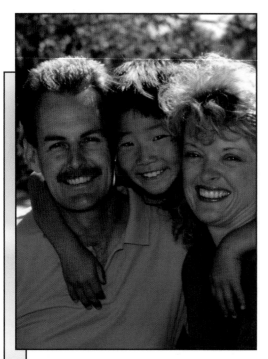

Adoption is a great solution to infertility for many couples. Tens of thousands of children are adopted every year in the United States.

Of course, many people who are unable to conceive decide to adopt children from someone else or from an agency. Others may decide that adoption is not right for them. They may come to realize that life without children of their own is OK. Many people, even those who are fertile, decide not to have children. These people can still be involved in children's lives, whether it's through volunteer work, as a teacher, camp counselor, or babysitter, or as a midwife or pediatrician. There are countless ways to make children a part of one's life.

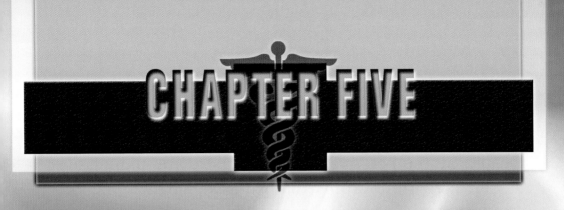

CHAPTER FIVE

Coping Strategies

oping with any kind of sexual health problem can be hard, but infertility may be especially difficult. In some parts of the world, people who are unable to have children are treated as outcasts. For cultural or religious reasons, these people are seen as misfits or mistakes. If they can't reproduce, the reasoning goes, then what is the point of their being here?

Fortunately, it's not like this in most places. Rather, infertility is looked at either as a fact of life that was just meant to be or as a treatable medical condition. As you now know, there are all kinds of ways to enable infertile couples to have children. Thanks to modern technology, as well as more conventional approaches such as adoption, almost anyone can experience parenthood. There are limitations, of course—especially financial ones. Infertility treatment is never cheap. But overall, in most cases, just the fact that someone is infertile does not prevent her or him from becoming a parent.

MENTAL AND EMOTIONAL STRESS

Despite all the potential solutions, there are many issues associated with infertility that would be challenging to almost anyone. There's the emotional trauma of finding out that you're infertile when you've dreamed of giving birth and raising your own children all your life. Relationship problems can arise, too. It's never easy when a couple that is trying to get pregnant discovers that one of them is infertile while the other is in perfect reproductive health. Couples who choose to undergo fertility treatment may be subjected to various tests and procedures, all of which can be emotionally and physically exhausting. Those who decide to adopt are similarly subjected to scrutiny, including all kinds of tests intended to ensure that they'll make good parents. In the end, many of those coping with

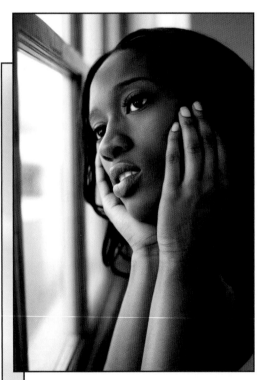

Finding out that you are infertile can cause sadness and confusion. Sometimes, just accepting your diagnosis is the most difficult part.

infertility face incredible stress. It's no easy task meeting the challenges of infertility.

HOTLINES AND SUPPORT GROUPS

Infertility can be especially difficult for those who don't have close friends or family to support them. They may experience intense loneliness and get the overwhelming feeling that no one understands or cares. Fortunately for these people, there are two great sources of help: hotlines and support groups.

Hotlines are usually toll-free telephone numbers. When you call, whoever picks up is knowledgeable about a particular disease or condition. The person on the other end of the line is there to help. Hotline operators can talk to the caller one-on-one, listen to his or her worries and concerns, and point the caller toward more information if necessary. There are no public national infertility hotlines. (Typically, the national hotlines are associated with corporations that make fertility drugs.) However, many local fertility clinics have staff available that can answer questions. One place to start is the local Planned Parenthood clinic. Planned Parenthood is a nonprofit group that helps people with family planning, including prevention of unwanted pregnancies and STDs. It also has information about fertility and infertility.

Two well-known hotlines for general information on sexual health are the National Women's Health Information

Center at (800) 994-9662 and the National Institute of Child Health and Human Development at (800) 370-2943. The American Social Health Association (800) 227-8922 is another good source of general information.

Support groups, on the other hand, are made up of people who come together to discuss their shared challenges and concerns. Many support groups are local. They might include five or ten individuals who gather once or twice a week in a church basement, a member's

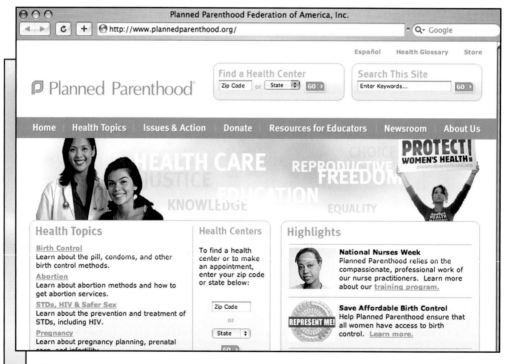

Planned Parenthood is a great resource for all things related to sex and sexual health. You can find a clinic in your area by looking in the phone book, or you can visit the Web site at www.plannedparenthood.org.

living room, or a community space such as a town hall or high school classroom. In general, an infertility support group would include men and women, singles and couples, who are seeking help and encouragement from people like themselves. A typical meeting might include time to share stories about emotional challenges, progress or setbacks, and successful treatments. Each person has a story to tell. That's the point of a support group. It is a place to share with, and listen to, compassionate members of the community.

Internet-based support groups are also popular. Infertility message boards, blogs, online forums, and listservs are all great ways to get information and support. Members can interact with each other through e-mail or by posting messages directly to Web sites. One such group is FertilityForums.com (part of FertilityCommunity.com).

People interested in adoption can find information online as well. Adoption.com is one good resource.

PREVENTATIVE HEALTH SCREENINGS

Sexually transmitted diseases (STDs) are a common cause of infertility. It's important that they be diagnosed and treated early, before they cause serious complications. STD screenings are one effective way to accomplish this.

Usually conducted by medical clinics, STD screenings are intended for sexually active individuals who believe they are at risk for contracting STDs. These individuals may include people who have recently had sex without using a barrier form of birth control (like a condom) that would reduce the risk of STDs.

The U.S. Centers for Disease Control and Prevention recommends annual screenings for certain individuals. These individuals include sexually active women ages twenty-five and younger, as well as all women who have new or multiple sex partners. These women should be tested, even if they show no sign of disease. The STDs that are the most dangerous when it comes to fertility

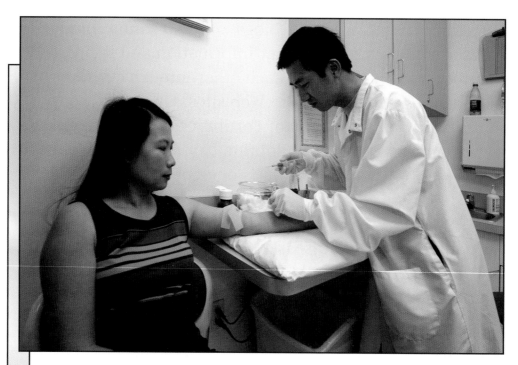

Testing for sexually transmitted diseases is often as simple as drawing blood and sending it off to a lab. Results usually come quickly—in a matter of days.

are chlamydia and gonorrhea. Infection with either of these bacteria can lead to pelvic inflammatory disease (PID), which in turn can cause complications including infertility. Screening for STDs is one of the keys to early detection, which means that treatment can begin before serious complications develop. A known carrier of an STD should take extra precautions to avoid spreading it to other people. Carriers should abstain from sexual contact, for instance, while their infection is active.

It's important to note that an STD screening that comes back negative (indicating no STD) does not mean it's now safe to have unprotected sex. STDs can be contracted at any time. One can never be entirely certain that his or her sex partner is not carrying an STD.

DOCTOR'S VISITS

Family physicians are a great resource when it comes to information on infertility and difficulties getting pregnant. They are also very knowledgeable about STDs and other conditions that might lead to infertility. If there is a health problem related to fertility, then your health care provider will know about it.

Some doctors are infertility specialists. They receive special training on treatment techniques and other ways of coping with infertility. Reproductive endocrinologists, for example, are doctors specializing in the function of hormones. (Hormones are crucial to fertility.) Reproductive endocrinologists work with both men and women. Obstetrician/gynecologists work with women. Urologists, on the other hand, focus on issues related to male reproduction.

An important part of any doctor's visit, whether it's for a routine checkup or a particular condition, is confidentiality. Physicians are required to maintain confidentiality regarding everything they learn about individuals who come to their office. Privacy is a priority. You can be

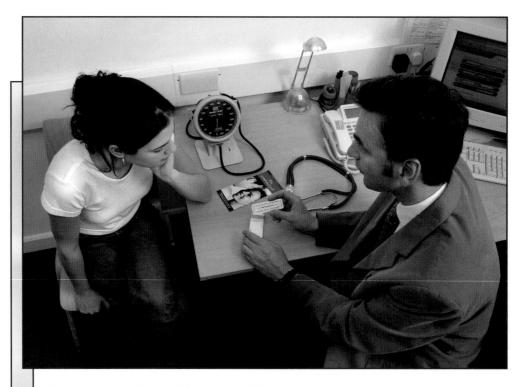

Your doctor or other health care provider can give you advice on contraception and safe sex. It's important to enter any sexual relationship cautiously, especially when it comes to STD prevention.

sure that what you say in the doctor's office will not leave the clinic.

The idea behind privacy, in part, is to enable patients to develop strong and open relationships with their health care providers. It's critical to be able to talk about anything—including STDs and other issues relevant to sexual health.

EDUCATION AND AWARENESS

Individuals with any disease or condition, including infertility, can benefit greatly by educating themselves as much as possible. As far as infertility is concerned, reading this book is a great start. But there are many other places to turn to as well. Textbooks, online resources, and even classroom discussions are all good sources of information about reproduction, fertility, and infertility.

Education and awareness are important when it comes to sexual health in general. The more you know, the more likely you can stay healthy. You'll be able to quickly recognize if things do go wrong and contact a doctor or other health professional for help.

HELPING A FRIEND

Infertility tends to be a very personal subject. Chances are you won't know if a friend or acquaintance is infertile and trying to cope. Furthermore, since he or she is likely to be older than you are (at least old enough to want to have children), it may not be appropriate to get involved.

Still, if you do have a friend who is coping with the challenges of infertility, one of the best things that you can do is listen. Good listeners take the time to sit down and allow their friend to open up. They don't offer advice. They just listen and attempt to understand.

Beyond just being there with open arms and open ears, it's possible to help others by sharing whatever knowledge you have. If you know about a clinic in the area that works with infertile individuals or couples, then pass along the information. If you know of other resources, then share them. Again, consider the circumstances before getting involved in another person's problems. In some cases, your help will be greatly appreciated. But in others, it's best to show your consideration by just being a friend.

Ten Great Questions to Ask Your Doctor

1. How would I know if I'm infertile?

2. Will problems I'm having now (with hormones, menstrual cycle, etc.) affect my fertility later?

3. Should I really be concerned about my fertility if I'm not planning to have children anytime soon?

4. Does my health now matter when it comes to future fertility?

5. What can I do now to improve my overall health?

6. Do I have any health conditions that would lead you to worry about my fertility?

7. Let's say I am infertile. What are my options for treatment?

8. Are there any side effects or possible dangers to these treatments?

9. Do you offer STD screening?

10. Are there support groups around for people coping with infertility?

GLOSSARY

artificial insemination Assistive reproductive technique that uses a syringe to place sperm in the uterus.

assistive reproductive technology (ART) Technology, like in vitro fertilization, that allows infertile people to have children.

conception Moment when an egg is fertilized by a sperm.

ejaculation Sudden discharge of semen.

endometrium The inner lining of the uterus, in which a fertilized egg embeds.

estrogen Female sex hormone produced primarily by the ovaries.

fallopian tubes Narrow passageways between the uterus and ovaries.

fertility Ability to conceive and carry a pregnancy to birth.

follicles Small sacs in the ovaries where eggs mature.

hormone Molecule released by endocrine glands into the blood; hormones serve as chemical messengers between cells.

infertile Unable to have children.

in vitro fertilization (IVF) Technique involving surgical removal of a woman's eggs, combining them with a man's sperm in the lab, and then transferring the fertilized eggs back into the woman's body.

laparoscopy Surgical technique using a thin, lighted instrument to observe and operate on organs within the abdomen.

menopause Period of life when a woman's menstrual cycle ceases.

menstruation Period; the phase of the menstrual cycle when bleeding occurs as the uterine lining is shed.

midwife A person who assists women in childbirth.

ovaries Female reproductive organs where eggs (ova) are produced.

ovulation Release of a mature egg (ovum) from the ovaries.

pathogenic Causing harm.

uterus Female organ where the fetus develops until birth; also called the womb.

zygote Fertilized egg.

FOR MORE INFORMATION

American College of Obstetricians and Gynecologists
P.O. Box 96920
Washington, DC 20090
(202) 638-5577
Web site: http://www.acog.org
This organization of medical professionals provides health
    care for women.

American Fertility Association
305 Madison Avenue, Suite 449
New York, NY 10165
(888) 917-3777
Web site: http://www.theafa.org
This national nonprofit organization provides information
    about infertility treatment and reproductive and
    sexual health.

American Social Health Association
P.O. Box 13827
Research Triangle Park, NC 27709
(919) 361-8400
Web site: http://www.ashastd.org

This nonprofit organization devoted to public health is an
authority on sexually transmitted disease information.

American Society for Reproductive Medicine
1209 Montgomery Highway
Birmingham, AL 35216-2809
(205) 978-5000
Web site: http://www.asrm.org
This nonprofit group is for medical professionals devoted
to reproductive health.

Health Canada
Address Locator 0900C2
Ottawa, ON K1A 0K9
Canada
(866) 225-0709
Web site: http://www.hc-sc.gc.ca
Health Canada is Canada's federal agency responsible for
helping citizens maintain and improve their health.

National Institutes of Health
9000 Rockville Pike
Bethesda, MD 20892
(301) 496-4000
Web site: http://www.nih.gov
Part of the U.S. Department of Health and Human Services,
the NIH is the primary federal agency for conducting

and supporting medical research, including studies on children's and teen's health.

Resolve: The National Infertility Association
8405 Greensboro Drive, Suite 800
McLean, VA 22102-5120
(703) 556-7172
Web site: http://www.resolve.org
This nonprofit organization promotes reproductive health and helps people with fertility disorders.

U.S. Centers for Disease Control and Prevention (CDC)
1600 Clifton Road
Atlanta, GA 30333
(800) CDC-INFO (232-4636)
Web site: http://www.cdc.gov/std
The CDC is the authoritative federal resource for information on all types of diseases and health-related issues.

WEB SITES

Due to the changing nature of Internet links, Rosen Publishing has developed an online list of Web sites related to the subject of this book. This site is updated regularly. Please use this link to access the list:

http://www.rosenlinks.com/lsh/fert

FOR FURTHER READING

Brynie, Faith Hickman. *101 Questions About Sex and Sexuality*. Minneapolis, MN: Twenty-First Century Books, 2003.

Cassan, A. *Human Reproduction and Development* (Inside the Human Body Series). New York, NY: Chelsea Clubhouse, 2005.

Hyde, Margaret O., and Elizabeth H. Forsyth. *Safe Sex 101: An Overview for Teens*. Minneapolis, MN: Twenty-First Century Books, 2006.

Parker, Steve. *The Reproductive System: Injury, Illness, and Health*. Chicago, IL: Heinemann Library, 2004.

Stanley, Deborah. *Sexual Health Information for Teens: Health Tips About Sexual Development, Human Reproduction, and Sexually Transmitted Diseases* (Teen Health Series). Detroit: MI, Omnigraphics, 2003.

Woods, Samuel G. *Everything You Need to Know About STD* (Sexually Transmitted Disease). New York, NY: Rosen Publishing Group, 2000.

BIBLIOGRAPHY

Campbell, Neil, Jane Reece, and Lawrence Mitchell. *Biology*. 5th ed. Menlo Park, CA: Benjamin/Cummings, 1999.

Ganong, William F. *Review of Medical Physiology*. 19th ed. Stamford, CT: Appleton & Lange, 1999.

MayoClinic.com. "Infertility." June 29, 2007. Retrieved February 29, 2008 (http://www.mayoclinic.com/health/infertility/DS00310/DSECTION = 3).

National Center for Health Statistics. "Fertility, Family Planning, and Women's Health." October 31, 2007. Retrieved February 29, 2008 (www.cdc.gov/nchs/products/pubs/pubd/series/sr23/pre-1/sr23_19.htm).

National Center for Health Statistics. "Infertility." October 31, 2007. Retrieved February 19, 2008 (http://www.cdc.gov/nchs/fastats/fertile.htm).

Tarkan, Laurie. "Lowering the Odds of Multiple Births." *New York Times*, February 19, 2008. Retrieved February 29, 2008 (http://www.nytimes.com/2008/02/19/health/19mult.html).

U.S. Centers for Disease Control and Prevention. "2005 Assisted Reproductive Technology (ART) Report: Home." December 12, 2007. Retrieved February 29, 2008 (http://www.cdc.gov/ART/ART2005).

Weiss, Deborah. "Pregnancy and Childbearing Among
U.S. Teens." Planned Parenthood. December 28, 2007.
Retrieved February 21, 2008 (www.plannedparenthood.
org/issues-action/sex-education/teen-pregnancy-
6239.htm).

INDEX

ABOUT THE AUTHOR

Michael R. Wilson is a health and science writer. He's written on many topics for Rosen Publishing, including the human brain, the cardiopulmonary system, the endrocrine system, pelvic inflammatory disease, and genetics.

PHOTO CREDITS

Designer: Nelson Sá; **Editor:** Christopher Roberts
Photo Researcher: Marty Levick